Conjunctivitis of the newborn

Prevention and treatment at the primary health care level

World Health Organization
Geneva
1986

ISBN 92 4 156088 6

© World Health Organization 1986

Publications of the World Health Organization enjoy copyright protection in accordance with the provisions of Protocol 2 of the Universal Copyright Convention. For rights of reproduction or translation of WHO publications, in part or *in toto*, application should be made to the Office of Publications, World Health Organization, Geneva, Switzerland. The World Health Organization welcomes such applications.

The designations employed and the presentation of the material in this publication do not imply the expression of any opinion whatsoever on the part of the Secretariat of the World Health Organization concerning the legal status of any country, territory, city or area or of its authorities, or concerning the delimitation of its frontiers or boundaries.

The mention of specific companies or of certain manufacturers' products does not imply that they are endorsed or recommended by the World Health Organization in preference to others of a similar nature that are not mentioned. Errors and omissions excepted, the names of proprietary products are distinguished by initial capital letters.

TYPESET IN INDIA
PRINTED IN ENGLAND

85/6445-Macmillan/Spottiswoode-8500

Contents

		Page
1.	**Introduction**	1
2.	**Review of available information related to conjunctivitis of the newborn**	2
	Causes	2
	Extent of the problem	3
	Data sources	3
	Review of available data	3
	Prophylaxis: current procedures and data on efficacy	5
	Silver nitrate	5
	Tetracycline	6
	Erythromycin	6
	Traditional practices	7
3.	**Diagnosis of conjunctivitis of the newborn**	8
	Clinical diagnosis	8
	Gonococcal conjunctivitis	8
	Chlamydial conjunctivitis	9
	Conjunctivitis due to other causes	9
	Laboratory diagnosis	10
	Smears and stains	10
	Culture methods	11
	Other techniques	11
4.	**Prevention strategies**	12
	Treatment of pregnant women	12
	Ocular prophylaxis in the newborn	13
	Silver nitrate solution	13
	Tetracycline hydrochloride eye ointment	13
	Recommendations	14

5. Treatment of manifest cases and exposed infants....... 15

    Treatment of gonococcal conjunctivitis of the newborn . 15
        Topical treatment............................ 15
        Systemic treatment........................... 16
    Treatment of presumed chlamydial and other non-gonococcal conjunctivitis of the newborn.......... 16
    Infants exposed to gonorrhoea 17

6. Health education and training of personnel 18

    Educational needs.............................. 18
    Training needs of health personnel 18

7. Logistics of supply of drugs....................... 20

8. Surveillance techniques and reporting................ 21

Acknowledgements...................................... 22

Summary... 23

Annex 1. Laboratory methods used for identifying causes of conjunctivitis of the newborn............... 24

Annex 2. Therapeutic recommendations for treatment of gonococcal infections in adults................ 28

Annex 3. List of participants........................ 30

1. Introduction

Purulent conjunctivitis of the newborn caused by *Neisseria gonorrhoeae* is a serious and potentially blinding condition, well known in most parts of the world. After the introduction in 1880 of Credé's preventive method, consisting of the instillation of silver nitrate drops into the eyes of the newborn child, the incidence of gonococcal conjunctivitis of the newborn decreased substantially in many countries, particularly where legislation and availability of health services enabled this prophylaxis to be applied systematically on a large scale. Nevertheless, in many countries where the incidence of gonorrhoea is high and where prophylaxis is not widely practised, conjunctivitis of the newborn is a health problem of growing importance, particularly since the emergence of penicillinase-producing strains of *N. gonorrhoeae* (PPNG).

The emergence of resistant strains of *N. gonorrhoeae* and the realization that *Chlamydia trachomatis* is another major cause of conjunctivitis of the newborn have led to changes in methods of prevention and treatment. Within the context of primary health care, it is important that more attention should be paid to the prevention and management of purulent conjunctivitis of the newborn: in this respect, personnel working at the community level, such as community health workers and traditional birth attendants, have a particularly important role in preventing blindness.

A WHO Working Group on the Prevention and Treatment of Ophthalmia Neonatorum at the Primary Level met in Geneva from 29 November to 2 December 1983 to address this issue and propose appropriate guidelines for intervention.[1]

Definition: conjunctivitis of the newborn is defined as any conjunctivitis with discharge occurring during the first 28 days of life. Other terms used for this disease include ophthalmia neonatorum, blennorrhoea neonatorum, and neonatal conjunctivitis. In this book, conjunctivitis of the newborn includes all these terms.

---

[1] The participants in the Working Group are listed in Annex 3.

2. Review of available information related to conjunctivitis of the newborn

Causes

The most serious cause of conjunctivitis of the newborn is *Neisseria gonorrhoeae*. Eye disease produced by this sexually transmitted organism is very obvious and may rapidly cause blindness; *N. gonorrhoeae* also causes systemic infections, particularly severe septicaemia.

Another important cause of conjunctivitis of the newborn is *Chlamydia trachomatis*. This organism can also be sexually transmitted and, like *N. gonorrhoeae*, causes genital-tract infection of the mother and infects the infant during its passage through the birth canal; however, chlamydial eye infections are less threatening to sight than gonococcal infections. Apart from the eye, *C. trachomatis* may infect other sites, such as the nasopharynx, and may cause pneumonia.

Other common causes of conjunctivitis of the newborn include *Staphylococcus aureus*, *Streptococcus pneumoniae*, *Haemophilus* spp., *Pseudomonas* spp., and occasionally other Gram-negative bacteria. The infections they cause are often hospital acquired and usually do not endanger sight.

In developing countries *N. gonorrhoeae* still accounts for 20–75% of cases of neonatal conjunctivitis, and *C. trachomatis* causes 15–35%. Strains of *N. gonorrhoeae* resistant to penicillin have become widespread in some areas, and consequently this antibiotic has become less useful for treatment.

In industrialized countries *C. trachomatis* is a more frequent cause of neonatal conjunctivitis than *N. gonorrhoeae*. Where prophylaxis is not performed, 1–15% of cases coming to medical attention are caused by *N. gonorrhoeae* and 25–50% by *C. trachomatis*. The remaining 35–74% are due to other causes or are of unknown cause; in the majority of these cases no microbial pathogen can be demonstrated.

2. REVIEW OF AVAILABLE INFORMATION

Extent of the problem

Data sources

The frequency and distribution of conjunctivitis of the newborn and its complications, particularly blindness, can be measured or estimated by using four different types of data.

(1) *Prevalence of gonococcal or chlamydial infections in pregnant women.* The risk of gonococcal and chlamydial neonatal conjunctivitis, in the absence of prophylaxis, can be estimated from the prevalence of genital infection in pregnant women and the transmission rates to newborn infants (30% for *N. gonorrhoeae* and 25–50% for *C. trachomatis*).

(2) *Consultation rates.* The rates of consultation for conjunctivitis of the newborn at different levels within the health service are significantly influenced by the use of prophylaxis; information on application of prophylaxis is therefore necessary for their interpretation. Few countries have a reporting system that includes data on conjunctivitis of the newborn and thus reliable data on the demand for treatment are generally lacking.

(3) *Cohort studies.* The incidence of conjunctivitis of the newborn (number of cases per 1000 live births) caused by gonococcal or chlamydial infections (or other causes) can be determined accurately by screening all children from consecutive births.

(4) *Prevalence of blindness.* In developing countries, data on blindness in children under 5 years old, and on the proportion caused by neonatal conjunctivitis, are seldom available. Where figures are available, they often indicate a low prevalence of blindness because it is associated with high mortality in early childhood; thus, in developing countries, gonococcal conjunctivitis may be a substantial health problem despite the apparent low prevalence of blindness.

Review of available data

Prevalence of gonococcal or chlamydial infections in pregnant women

The prevalence of sexually transmitted diseases has been increasing throughout the world for the past three decades. Not only is the incidence of gonorrhoea currently at a very high level, but there is direct and indirect evidence that *C. trachomatis* infections are becoming increasingly common. The prevalence of these infections among pregnant women is particularly important because they cause maternal complications and serious disease, including conjunctivitis, in the neonate.

Data on infection levels during pregnancy are incomplete, but *N. gonorrhoeae* can be recovered from 4-18% of pregnant women in some developing countries, and from 0.1-7% in industrialized countries with well-developed health services. It is known that about 30% of infants exposed to *N. gonorrhoeae* during birth will develop gonococcal infection of the eye if prophylaxis is not given; this implies that up to about 6% of infants born in some developing countries will develop gonococcal conjunctivitis.

The corresponding figures for *C. trachomatis* infections are more difficult to determine because reliable laboratory facilities to detect this agent are not widely available. In the United States of America, *C. trachomatis* infection of the genital tract has been found in 2-24% of pregnant women. Between 25% and 50% of neonates exposed to this infection during birth develop chlamydial conjunctivitis so that 0.5-12% of all newborn children may be infected depending on the population group. Data from the developing countries are incomplete, but up to 7% of pregnant women have been reported to have chlamydial infection in some populations.

Consultation rates

Estimates of incidence based on consultation rates are rare. In industrialized countries the incidence has been estimated as 0.4 per 1000 live births for gonococcal conjunctivitis and 1.1-4.4 per 1000 live births for chlamydial conjunctivitis. Corresponding data from developing countries for gonococcal conjunctivitis indicate an incidence of 10 cases per 1000 live births. The figures are, however, probably gross underestimates.

Cohort studies

In industrialized countries, the incidence of gonococcal conjunctivitis of the newborn is low, being 0.1-0.6 per 1000 live births. For chlamydial infections, studies in the United States of America have reported incidences ranging from 5 to 60 cases per 1000 live births, and one study in the United Kingdom reported an incidence of 4 per 1000 live births.

Prevalence of blindness

At the turn of the last century, 20-40% of children in European institutions for the blind were there as a result of gonococcal conjunctivitis of the newborn. However, since the introduction of silver nitrate prophylaxis, the number of children affected has continuously declined. For example, in the United Kingdom no cases of blindness due to conjunctivitis of the newborn have been reported since 1955.

There are no data available for developing countries on the proportion of blindness caused by conjunctivitis of the newborn. In these countries, blind children have a high mortality rate and, therefore, the prevalence of eye infection appears to be low.

Generally, data from developing countries are limited from each of the four sources reviewed, so that the prevalence of the condition is substantially underestimated.

Conjunctivitis of the newborn is becoming an increasingly serious health problem in developing countries for the following reasons:

—ocular prophylaxis is not available, has been discontinued, or is applied only to a small proportion of newborn infants;
—an increasing number of gonococcal infections are due to penicillin-resistant strains; and
—treatment for gonococcal conjunctivitis of the newborn is not generally available, and if the infection is caused by a penicillin-resistant strain treatment is often inadequate.

Prophylaxis: current procedures and data on efficacy

Silver nitrate

In the absence of systematic diagnosis and treatment of maternal genital infections before delivery, most cases of conjunctivitis of the newborn can be prevented by disinfection of the infant's conjunctivae immediately after birth. In its present form the Credé procedure has two components: (1) cleaning of the infant's eyelids and (2) the instillation of 1% silver nitrate solution into the conjunctival sacs. These measures must be carried out as soon as possible after birth, and can easily be done by traditional birth attendants and other community health workers.

Studies have shown that about 30% of babies exposed to infection during birth will develop gonococcal conjunctivitis if a preventive measure is not applied; this figure is reduced to 2% if silver nitrate prophylaxis is used. In populations with a high risk of gonococcal infection the value of silver nitrate prophylaxis has been well established. However, silver nitrate prophylaxis does not prevent conjunctivitis of the newborn that is caused by *C. trachomatis*.

Silver ions kill bacteria by binding to their surface proteins, but the preparation may irritate the conjunctiva. Up to 90% of infants show some signs of chemical conjunctivitis 3–6 hours after the application of 1% silver nitrate solution, but in most infants this subsides after 24 hours. Damage to the eye has occurred after the application of a silver nitrate solution that has become more concentrated through evaporation.

Although prophylaxis with silver nitrate has been very successful, some reservations have been expressed. At present, the objections to silver nitrate prophylaxis are: (1) it does not provide absolute protection against gonococcal conjunctivitis; (2) it has no effect against *C. trachomatis* infections, which are more common in some countries; and (3) it causes transient chemical conjunctivitis. On the other hand, silver nitrate solutions are widely available and inexpensive, and there is no evidence of resistance of *N. gonorrhoeae* strains.

Tetracycline

Ophthalmic solutions and ointments containing tetracycline have been used for the prophylaxis of neonatal conjunctivitis. The infant's eyes are carefully cleaned immediately after birth and a single application of 1% tetracycline hydrochloride is administered to the conjunctivae. Although tetracycline has proved to be effective in preventing gonococcal conjunctivitis of the newborn, there is disagreement as to whether it is more or less effective than silver nitrate. Some strains of *N. gonorrhoeae*, e.g., penicillinase-producing strains (PPNG) of east Asian origin, are resistant to tetracycline, but the significance of this for topical treatment or prophylaxis is not known. Studies to evaluate the efficacy of prophylaxis with topical tetracycline in areas with high levels of antibiotic resistance to gonococci should therefore be encouraged.

Tetracycline hydrochloride is active against *C. trachomatis*, but the results of its prophylactic use against chlamydial conjunctivitis of the newborn are not conclusive, and further studies are needed.

Erythromycin

When available, eye ointment containing erythromycin (0.5%) can be used as an alternative to silver nitrate or tetracycline. Although the results of only a few studies are available, it is probably as effective as tetracycline hydrochloride ointment against gonococcal conjunctivitis.

Erythromycin is active against *C. trachomatis*, but the results of its prophylactic use against chlamydial neonatal conjunctivitis are not conclusive, and further studies are needed.

2. REVIEW OF AVAILABLE INFORMATION

Traditional practices

In some regions, traditional "medications" (e.g., lemon juice, cooking oil, and mother's milk) are applied to the eyes of newborn infants. Some of these substances are irritants and may cause eye damage. Moreover, it is not known to what extent these traditional medications are effective against *N. gonorrhoeae* and *C. trachomatis*.

3. Diagnosis of conjunctivitis of the newborn

Clinical diagnosis

The clinical picture and course of conjunctivitis of the newborn depend on whether it is caused by *N. gonorrhoeae, C. trachomatis*, or other bacterial infections acquired at or after birth.

Although each etiological agent produces a slightly different pattern of disease, there is considerable overlap; therefore, identification of the infecting organism cannot be based on clinical signs alone. As a general rule, however, gonococcal eye infection tends to be more severe, of earlier onset, and is potentially blinding.

Fig. 1–13 show the clinical signs of conjunctivitis of the newborn caused by different organisms, and Fig. 14–17 show the histological features of gonococcal and chlamydial conjunctivitis.

Gonococcal conjunctivitis

Gonococcal conjunctivitis appears between 1 and 13 days after birth, usually by the third day; it is bilateral in most infants. The inflammation normally starts with hyperaemia and shedding of tears, followed about one day later by the appearance of a mucopurulent/purulent discharge which may contain blood. The eyelids become very swollen. The discharge is often profuse and under considerable pressure behind the lids so that medical personnel examining these infants should protect their own eyes from ejected discharge when the lids are forcibly opened for examination. The conjunctivae covering the anterior surface of the eyeballs become swollen with fluid and there is marked infiltration and swelling of the conjunctivae on the inner side of the lids. Severe inflammation may give rise to inflammatory membranes that bleed if an attempt is made to remove them; as the disease resolves, these membranes often result in scarring of the conjunctivae.

Corneal involvement first appears as diffuse epithelial oedema, which gives the cornea a hazy, greyish appearance. Coarse grey-white

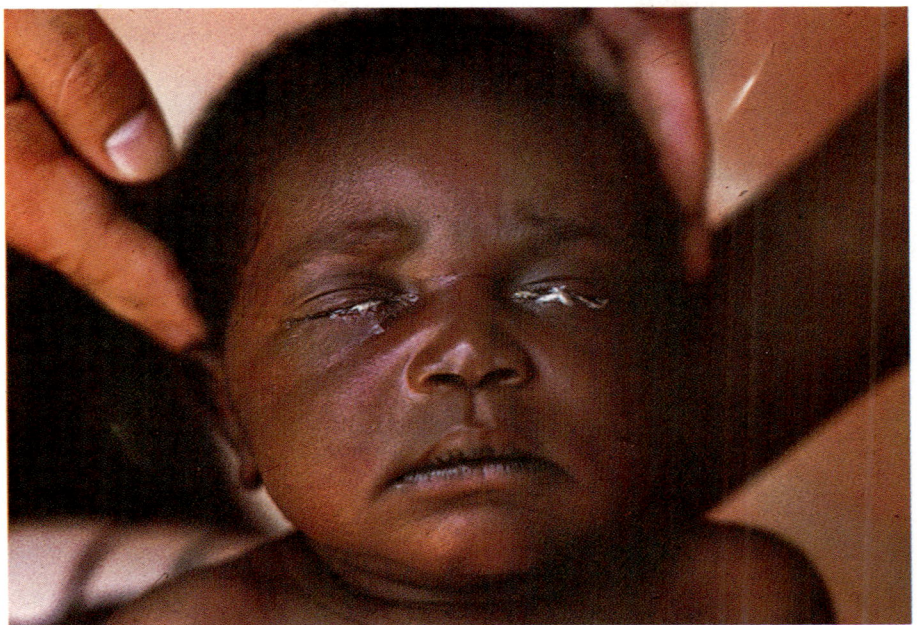

Fig. 1. A 12-day-old infant with bilateral gonococcal conjunctivitis.

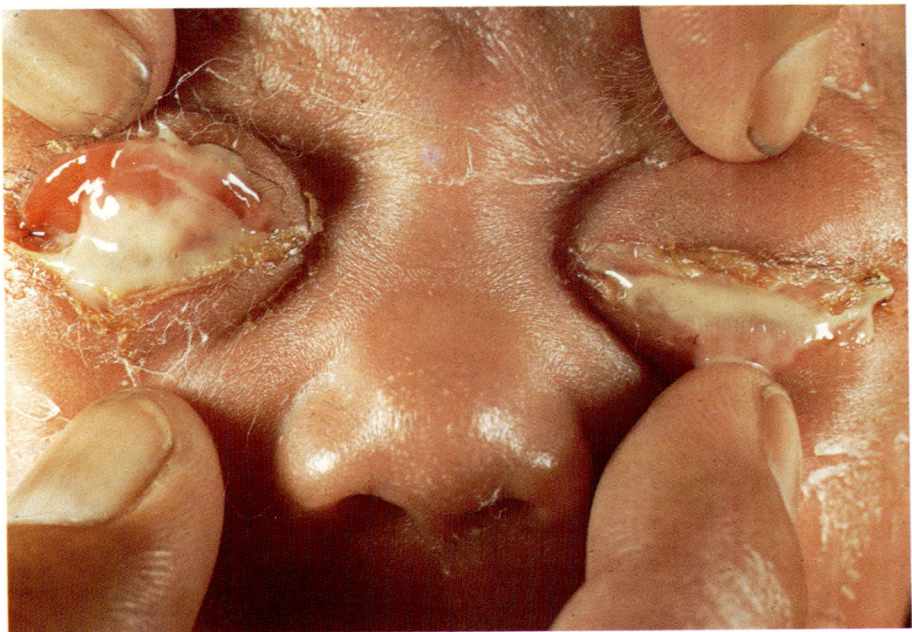

Fig. 2. A newborn infant with purulent conjunctivitis caused by *Neisseria gonorrhoeae*. The large amount of exudate is typical of gonococcal eye infection.

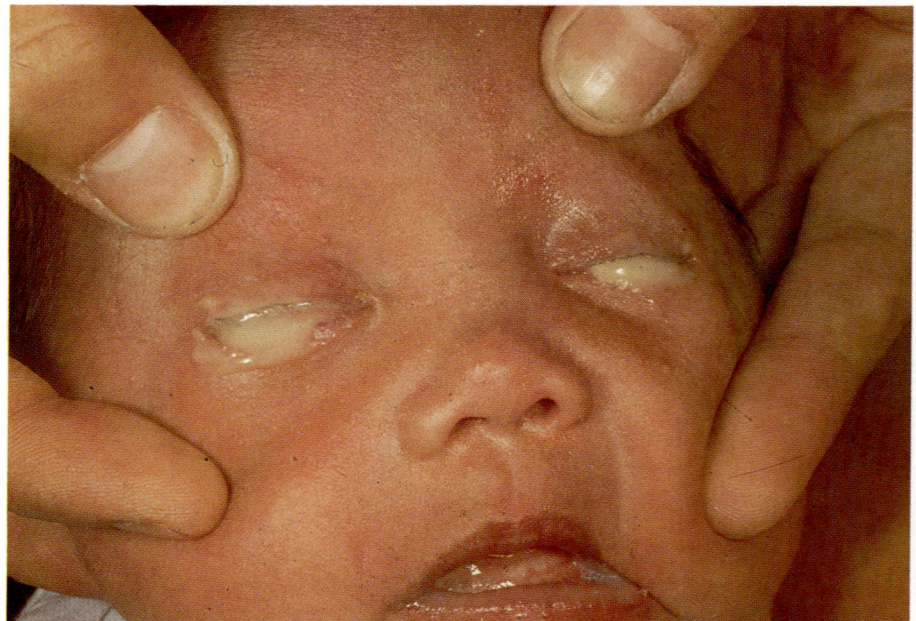

Fig. 3. A newborn infant with conjunctivitis caused by antibiotic-resistant *N. gonorrhoeae*.

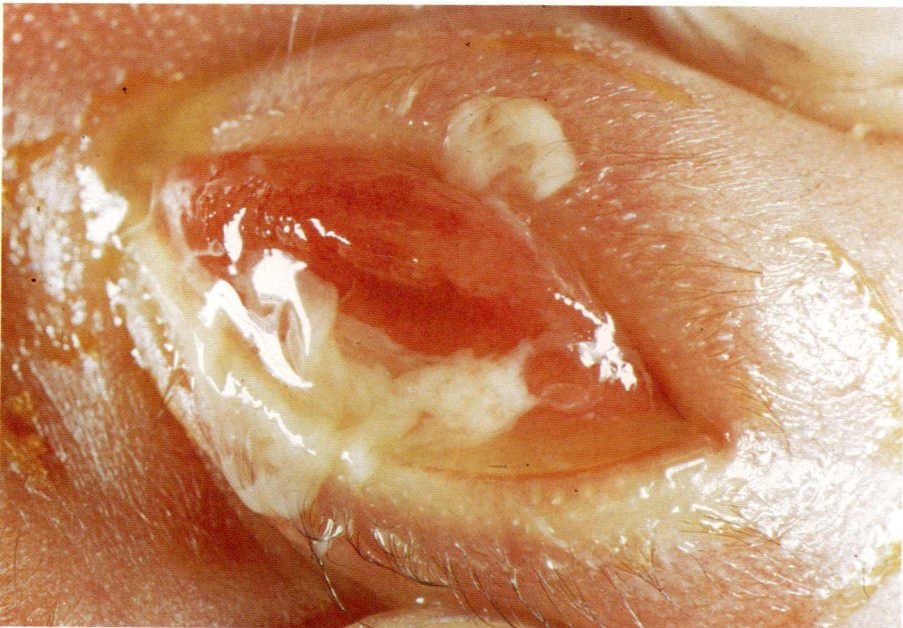

Fig. 4. The eye of a newborn infant with gonococcal conjunctivitis. The inflamed conjunctiva is infiltrated and swollen, so that it extrudes beyond the lid margin when the lower lid is pulled down. In such cases it is difficult to examine the cornea, which is hidden by inflamed conjunctiva and discharge.

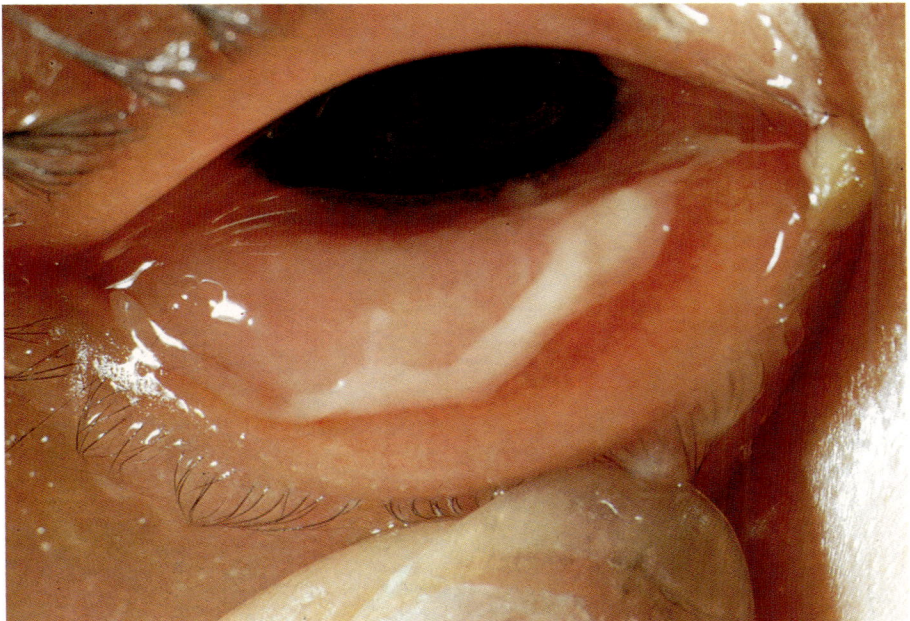

Fig. 5. An inflammatory membrane in an infant with conjunctivitis caused by *Haemophilus*. Inflammatory membranes are adherent to the conjunctivae, and if removed cause profuse bleeding. Membrane formation often results in scarring of the conjunctivae as the disease resolves.

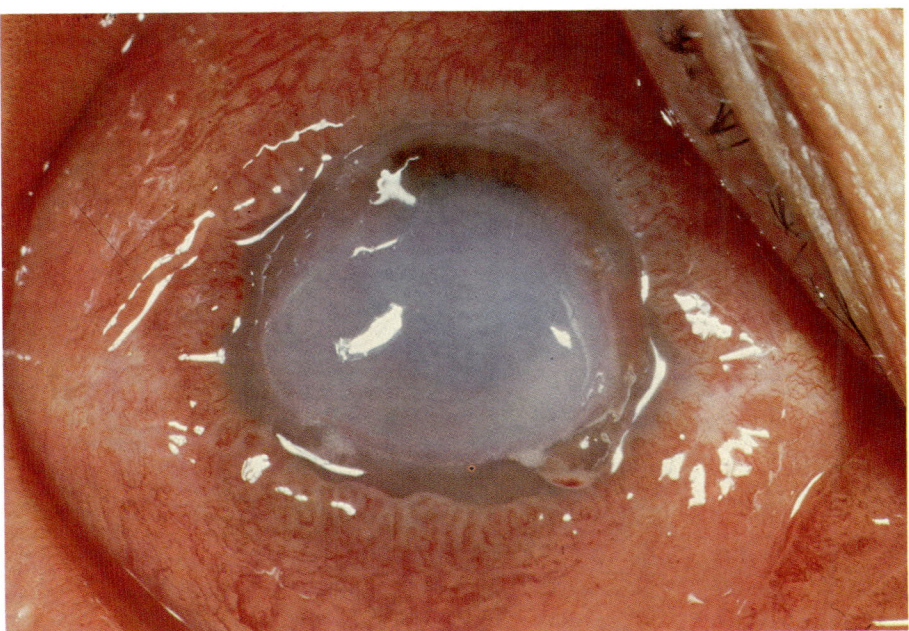

Fig. 6. Corneal ulceration and opacity caused by gonococcal conjunctivitis. Between the milky, opaque central cornea and the swollen, hyperaemic conjunctiva, the cornea has developed an ulcer and has become very thin; the brown iris lying underneath the cornea can easily be seen.

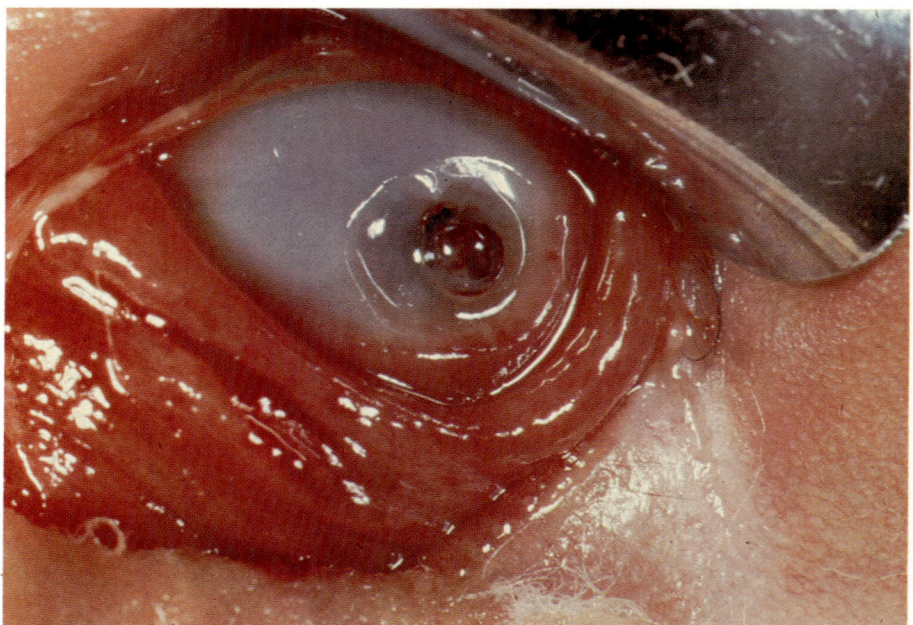

Fig. 7. Untreated gonococcal conjunctivitis in a 3-week-old infant. The cornea is opaque and a peripheral ulcer has developed which has perforated the cornea. The iris can be seen forming a plug at the base of the ulcer.

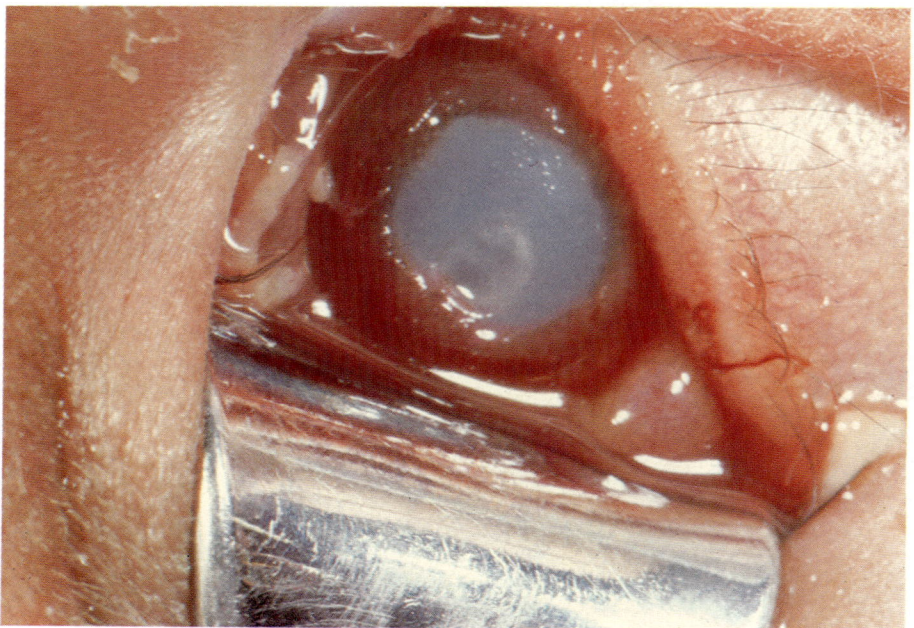

Fig. 8. Gonococcal conjunctivitis in a 2-month-old infant. The cornea is opaque and an ulcer may be seen at the bottom, which extends almost to the centre of the cornea. The conjunctiva is swollen and extremely inflamed.

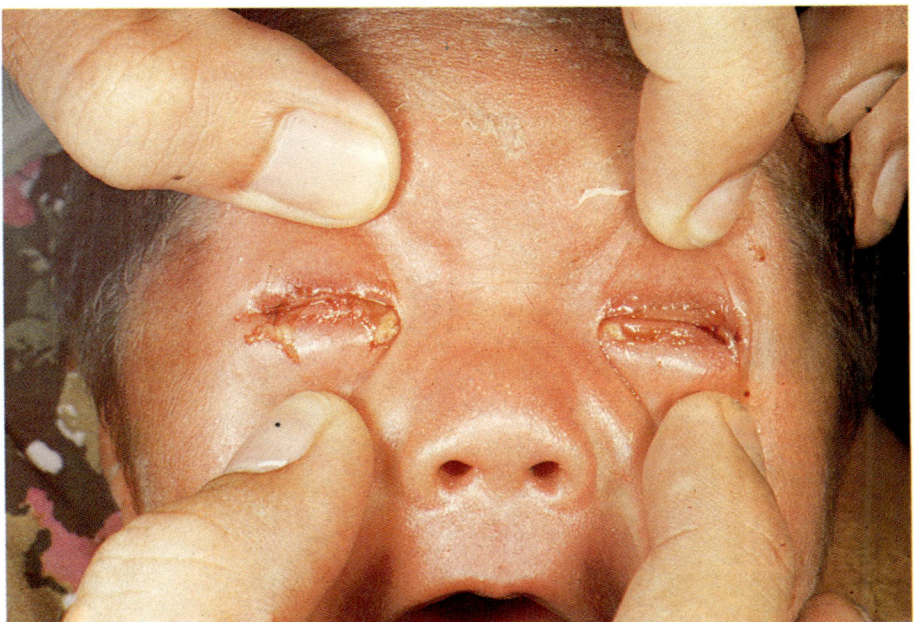

Fig. 9. A newborn infant with bilateral conjunctivitis caused by *Chlamydia trachomatis*. The discharge is usually less abundant in chlamydial conjunctivitis than in gonococcal conjunctivitis.

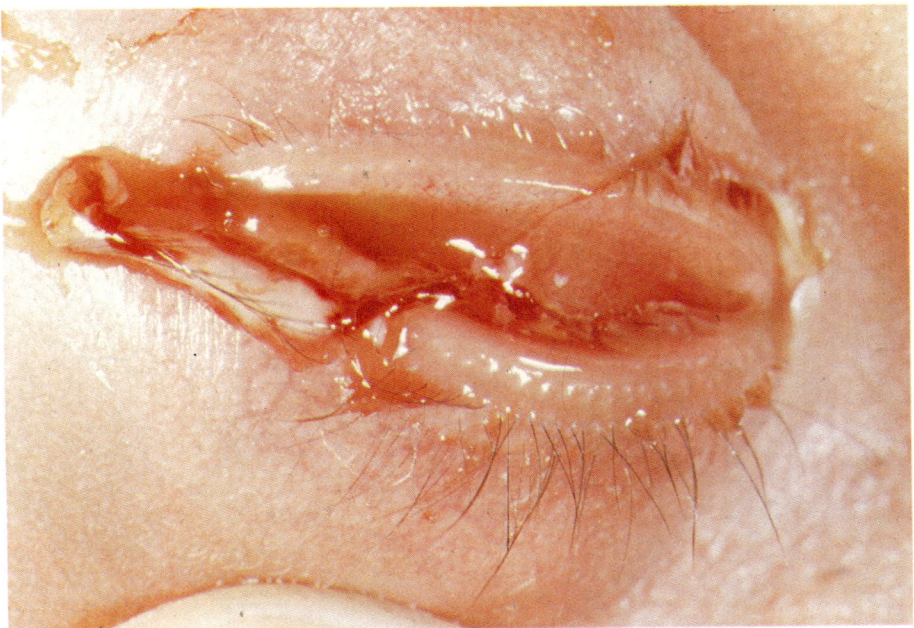

Fig. 10. Close-up view of the eye shown in Fig. 9 (chlamydial conjunctivitis). Blood staining of the discharge often occurs because the conjunctiva bleeds when the lid is pulled down for examination.

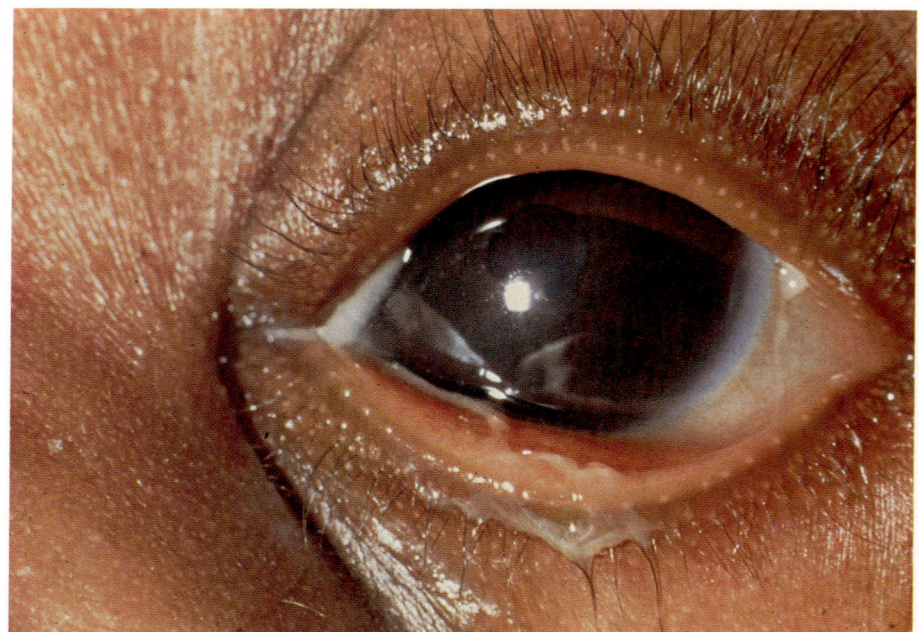

Fig. 11. Conjunctivitis caused by *Chlamydia trachomatis* in a newborn infant; there is only a small amount of ocular discharge.

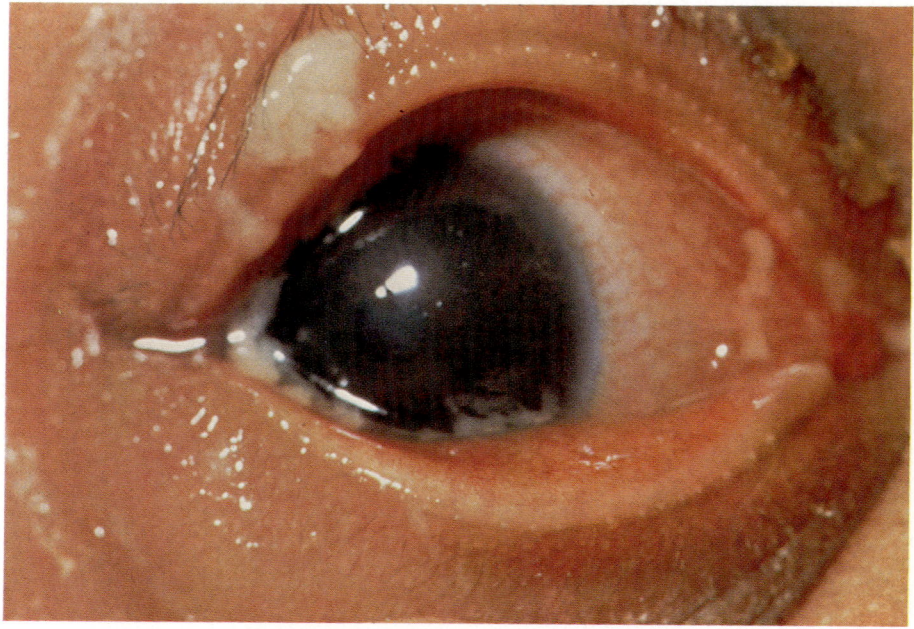

Fig. 12. Chlamydial conjunctivitis in a newborn infant.

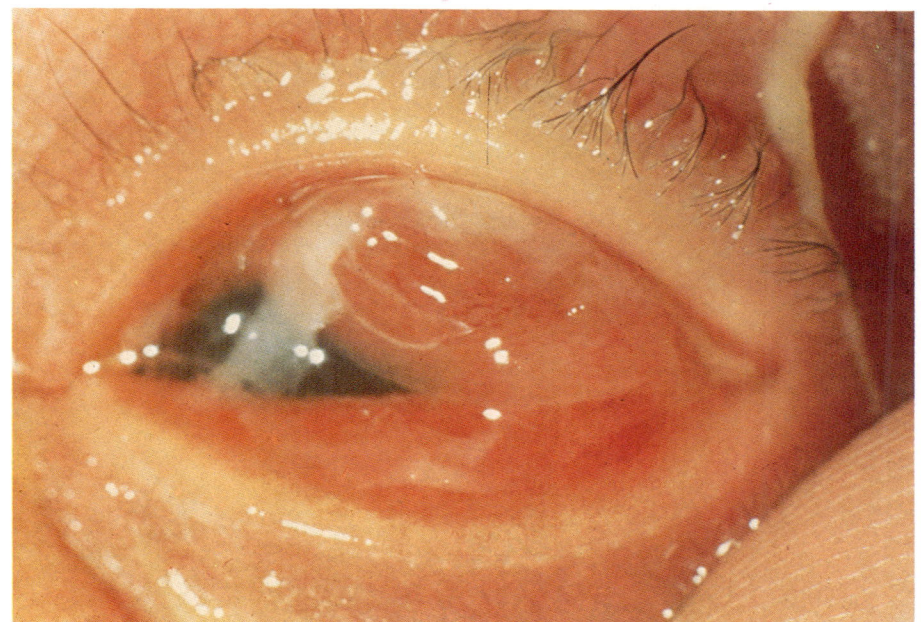

Fig. 13. Severe conjunctivitis caused by *Chlamydia trachomatis* in a newborn infant. The conjunctiva is markedly swollen and inflamed, and there is ocular discharge.

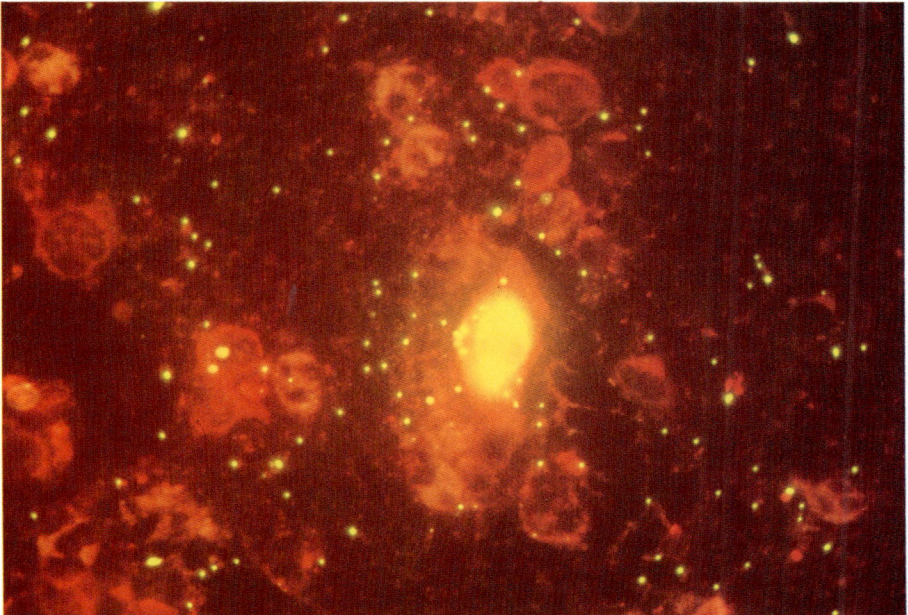

Fig. 14. Conjunctival scraping from a newborn infant showing a chlamydial inclusion in the centre, and many small bright particles (elementary bodies) scattered around. The specimen has been stained with anti-chlamydial monoclonal antibodies, labelled with fluorescein; inclusions and elementary bodies are shown as bright spots.

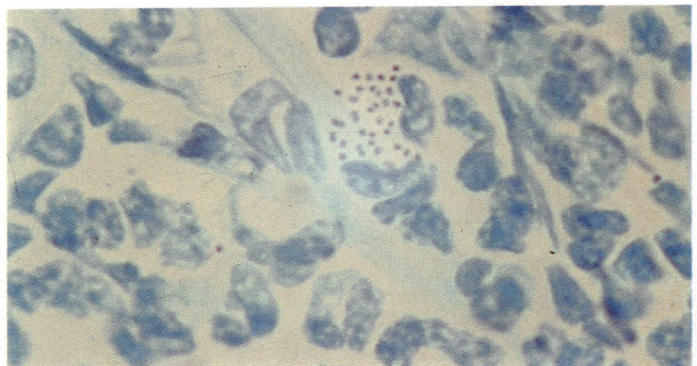

Fig. 15. Intracellular gonococci in a conjunctival smear stained with methylene blue.

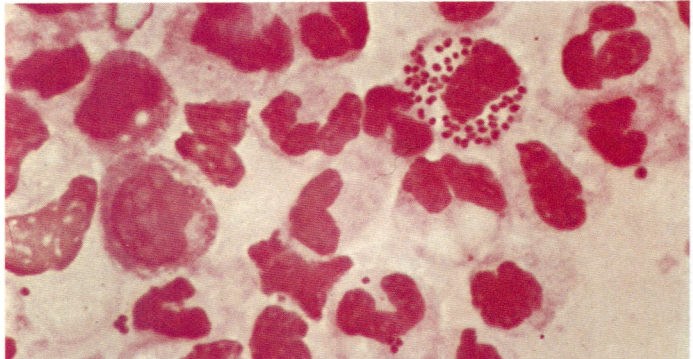

Fig. 16. Intracellular Gram-negative gonococci in a conjunctival smear stained with Gram stain.

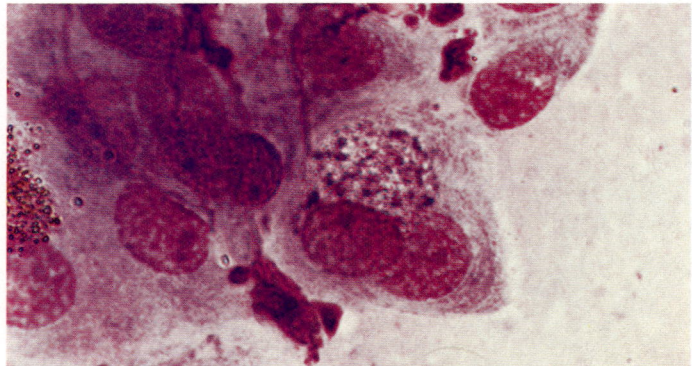

Fig. 17. Intracytoplasmic inclusions of *Chlamydia trachomatis* in a conjunctival scraping stained with Giemsa.

opacities (infiltrations) appear near the border of the cornea and the sclera during the second week of the disease. The infiltrations at the edge of the cornea enlarge and become ulcerated by the end of the second or during the third week; the centre of the cornea may also become ulcerated. Ulceration often progresses to perforation of the eyeball with loss of vision. From the fourth to the eighth week new blood vessels begin to invade the cornea, and corneal scarring may occur in infants with ulceration and perforation.

If untreated, gonococcal infection of the newborn may be associated with extra-ocular manifestations such as arthritis or septicaemia.

The severity of gonococcal conjunctivitis of the newborn varies considerably, and not all cases result in blindness. The initiation of treatment dramatically changes the course and outcome of the disease, usually with recognizable improvement within 24 hours. It is therefore extremely important that early treatment is given to prevent corneal complications. The application of topical steroids in any form may increase the likelihood of perforation of the cornea and therefore they should never be used in the treatment of neonatal conjunctivitis.

Chlamydial conjunctivitis

Chlamydial conjunctivitis characteristically appears between 5 and 14 days after birth. Approximately half the cases are bilateral. Inflammation usually starts with mucopurulent discharge and swelling of the eyelids; there is usually hyperaemia and swelling of the conjunctivae. In some infants, the conjunctivae bleed easily on examination. Inflammatory membranes may occur, usually during the second week of the disease. If the disease is active for more than four weeks, discrete nodules (lymphoid follicles) will appear in the conjunctivae. Unlike gonococcal conjunctivitis, blinding corneal complications are not associated with chlamydial infections. Possible extra-ocular manifestations include palpable pre-auricular lymph nodes, pneumonia, and otitis media.

With appropriate treatment, the ocular discharge usually disappears within two days, but inflammatory hypertrophy of the conjunctivae and the lymphoid follicles may persist for several weeks.

Conjunctivitis due to other causes

Conjunctivitis of the newborn may also be caused by various other bacteria, such as *Staphylococcus aureus, Streptococcus pneumoniae, Haemophilus* spp., *Pseudomonas* spp., and less frequently other Gram-negative bacteria. Discharge is usually present in these cases during the first week of life. However, the clinical signs and symptoms are usually very mild compared with those of gonococcal or chlamydial conjunctivitis. Swelling of the eyelids is usually minimal, but there may be slight conjunctival congestion. Corneal complications are extremely rare but have been reported in cases of *Pseudomonas* infection. Ocular infection with *Herpes simplex* virus is uncommon in the newborn.

Laboratory diagnosis[1]

At the primary health care level, conjunctivitis of the newborn is usually diagnosed clinically, because laboratory facilities are rarely available. If they are available, the diagnostic tests used will depend upon the level of resources.

Three levels of laboratory services are recognized. In peripheral laboratories, equipment and expertise are limited and the diagnosis of gonococcal eye infection is usually restricted to the examination of stained smears of conjunctival pus. Laboratories at the intermediate level are better equipped and should be able to use culture methods to diagnose gonococcal conjunctivitis. Central laboratories are generally well equipped and have highly trained staff and can therefore perform more sophisticated tests, such as the diagnosis of chlamydial infection using smears of epithelial cells scraped from the conjunctiva and stained by the Giemsa method. Central laboratories should also be able to detect penicillinase-producing strains of *N. gonorrhoeae* (PPNG).

Although laboratory methods are obviously useful for diagnosing individual cases of conjunctivitis of the newborn, they are also essential for epidemiological studies, e.g., for determining the distribution and prevalence of gonococcal isolates that are resistant to penicillin.

Resistant gonococcal strains can be differentiated into two groups: the penicillinase-producing *N. gonorrhoeae* (PPNG) strains, and chromosomally resistant strains. Studies of the resistance to other antibiotics (e.g., tetracycline and spectinomycin) should be encouraged since this information is necessary for planning the best strategies for control at the national level.

Smears and stains

Gonococcal infection

The basic laboratory technique for diagnosing gonococcal infection is the examination of a stained swab smear of conjunctival exudate.

---

[1] Specific details of various diagnostic methods are given in Annex 1.

The best stain for indentifying *N. gonorrhoeae* is Gram stain, but methylene blue is a good alternative. Smears should be reported as positive when typical intracellular Gram-negative diplococci are found; as inconclusive (equivocal) if only atypical or extracellular diplococci are present; and as negative if no diplococci are present.

Chlamydial infection

Where a well-equipped laboratory with experienced staff is available, the diagnostic method of choice for chlamydial eye infections is the microscopic examination of a smear of epithelial cells scraped from the conjunctiva and stained by the Giemsa method. Intracytoplasmic inclusions of *C. trachomatis* can be identified only in intact conjunctival epithelial cells. Such cells are not found in smears of pus or exudate and can only be obtained by scraping the surface of the conjunctiva. Clearly this is not a diagnostic technique that is widely applicable at the primary health care level.

Culture methods

Gonococcal infection

If appropriate facilities are available, *N. gonorrhoeae* can be isolated by culture techniques. A variety of culture media can be used, e.g., Thayer-Martin medium, enriched chocolate agar, or sheep's (but not human) blood agar. If the isolation medium cannot be inoculated immediately, the sample of conjunctival discharge should be transferred to a transport medium such as Transgrow[1] or Stuart medium.

Chlamydial infection

When available, procedures for the identification of *Chlamydia* by culture are usually limited to central laboratories. The techniques required (cell culture, etc.) are similar to those required for virus isolation.

Other techniques

For both *N. gonorrhoeae* and *C. trachomatis*, research is proceeding to develop rapid, simple, and inexpensive methods for antigen recognition, e.g., the use of fluorescein-labelled monoclonal antibodies for detecting *C. trachomatis*, and enzyme-activated tests for both *Chlamydia* and *N. gonorrhoeae*.

---

[1] Martin, J. E. & Lester, A. Transgrow, a medium for transport and growth of *Neisseria gonorrhoeae* and *Neisseria meningitidis*. HMSHA Health Reports, **86**(1): 30 (1971).

4. Prevention strategies

Treatment of pregnant women

Ideally, primary prevention of gonococcal or chlamydial conjunctivitis of the newborn is best achieved by identifying and treating infected pregnant women. Pregnant women who are known to have gonococcal infection or who have had recent sexual contact with an infected partner should receive full treatment against gonorrhoea. One of the recommended treatments for these women and their sexual partners in areas where penicillin-resistant gonococci comprise less than 1% of isolates is aqueous procaine benzylpenicillin, 4.8 g (4.8 million IU) given by intramuscular injection, with 1 g of probenecid (if available) by mouth. In areas where penicillin-resistant gonococci are more frequent, a recommended treatment is 2 g of spectinomycin given by intramuscular injection.

More comprehensive recommendations for treatment of gonococcal infections were adopted at the sixth meeting of the WHO Expert Committee on Venereal Diseases and Treponematoses which was held in Geneva from 1 to 7 November 1983. These recommendations are given in Annex 2.

In most countries, screening of all pregnant women is either impracticable or not sufficiently cost-effective. This is particularly true for genital chlamydial infection because present diagnostic techniques are complex and expensive. However, it may be feasible to screen pregnant women in high-risk groups, including:

—pregnant women who have had recent sexual contact with a partner with an unspecified sexually transmitted disease;
—pregnant women with recent symptoms of sexually transmitted disease, such as vaginal discharge or dysuria;
—pregnant women with any other sexually transmitted disease such as syphilis, genital herpes, genital warts, or pubic lice; and
—women in their first pregnancy and without a steady partner.

Under ideal circumstances, screening should consist of separate culture of specimens taken from the cervix, rectum, and urethra; however, screening can be limited to culture of a cervical specimen alone. Screening of high-risk groups should be carried out wherever facilities are available and treatment started as early as possible in pregnancy; sexual partners should also be treated. Screening should be repeated in the last weeks of pregnancy.

Ocular prophylaxis in the newborn

Prophylaxis prevents most cases of gonococcal conjunctivitis of the newborn. Systematic detection and treatment of infected mothers are not available in many areas and therefore the application of prophylactic measures to the newborn child is often the only means of reducing the incidence of this potentially blinding disease.

Prophylaxis involves careful cleaning of the eyes immediately after birth, followed by the application of an antiseptic or antimicrobial agent to the conjunctivae. No perfect medication exists for this purpose, but the two main choices are 1% silver nitrate eye drops, and 1% tetracycline hydrochloride eye ointment. Erythromycin (0.5%) eye ointment is an alternative prophylactic agent, but it is not widely available.

Silver nitrate solution

Advantages:
1. It is active against all strains of *N. gonorrhoeae*, regardless of their antibiotic susceptibility.
2. It is inexpensive and widely available.
3. It is easy to apply.

Disadvantages:
1. It often causes a transient chemical conjunctivitis. The solution may cause ocular damage if it becomes too concentrated through evaporation; this can be prevented by dispensing it in small containers, avoiding prolonged storage, or using single-dose preparations.
2. It is ineffective in preventing chlamydial conjunctivitis of the newborn.

Tetracycline hydrochloride eye ointment

Advantages:
1. It is active against most strains of *N. gonorrhoeae*, and against *C. trachomatis*.
2. It is inexpensive and widely available.
3. It does not cause significant chemical conjunctivitis.

Disadvantages:
1. Some strains of *N. gonorrhoeae* are resistant to tetracycline (but topical application of tetracycline may overcome this resistance).

2. It may be difficult to introduce the ointment into the conjunctival sac.
3. It may be more expensive than silver nitrate, and it is not always available or properly stored.

Recommendations

There is no doubt that the best way to prevent neonatal conjunctivitis is to diagnose and treat maternal infections before delivery. This implies that all pregnant women, or at least those who have a high risk of contracting a sexually transmitted disease, should be screened. However, large-scale screening procedures may not be practicable and, because they are expensive, their use in low-risk populations cannot be justified.

In areas where the risk of gonococcal infection is high, the eyelids of every newborn child should be cleaned as soon as possible after birth and 1% silver nitrate eye drops applied. As an alternative, 1% tetracycline hydrochloride ointment can be used. Repeated doses of silver nitrate should not be given for either prophylaxis or treatment of conjunctivitis.

In areas where the risk of gonococcal infection is low, but where chlamydial infection is frequent (e.g., some industrialized countries), certain countries have chosen not to use any form of prophylaxis. However, the prophylactic use of 1% tetracycline ointment or, if available, 0.5% erythromycin ointment is preferable under such circumstances.

5. Treatment of manifest cases and exposed infants

Treatment of gonococcal conjunctivitis of the newborn

Conjunctivitis of the newborn that starts within the first week of life or that has a purulent discharge should be presumed to be of gonococcal origin, and treated as such. If the infection is mild or of late onset, a smear of conjunctival exudate may be useful to detect *N. gonorrhoeae*. If the infant has received previous treatment of any kind other than prophylaxis, this laboratory test may not be reliable. In these circumstances, the decision to treat a case as gonococcal conjunctivitis will depend on the clinical signs alone.

All cases of presumed gonococcal conjunctivitis must be treated with both an effective systemic *and* a topical antimicrobial agent; while topical treatment is essential, it should not be used alone. However, if a patient has to be referred for systemic treatment, topical treatment should be started immediately.

Topical treatment

The eyes must be cleaned before a topical antibiotic preparation can be applied. Tetracycline hydrochloride (1 %) ointment is the preferred medication, but 0.5 % erythromycin eye ointment can be used.

To remove discharge from the eye, the lids should be wiped with a moist clean cloth or cotton wool, or irrigated with saline or cooled, boiled water. Immediately after cleaning the eye, the antibiotic should be applied by pulling down the lower lid and placing the ointment on the exposed conjunctiva. Care should be taken to keep the ointment in the eye when the lid is released.

Topical treatment should be repeated every hour for the first 24 hours. During the second day, the eye should be treated 8 times. When the discharge and swelling have diminished, treatment can be reduced to 4 times a day, but should be continued for a total of 10 days. The mother of the child should be taught how to clean the eyes and to apply the ointment before leaving the health centre or hospital.

Systemic treatment

To achieve maximum efficacy, prompt treatment with systemic antibiotics is essential for every suspected case of gonococcal conjunctivitis of the newborn.

In areas where the prevalence of penicillin-resistant gonococci is known to be less than 1%, it is justifiable to treat gonococcal conjunctivitis of the newborn with penicillin. The recommended dosage of benzylpenicillin is 30 mg/kg (50 000 units/kg) given intramuscularly in 2 divided doses per day for 3 days. This should be accompanied by topical application of tetracycline or erythromycin eye ointment.

If the prevalence of penicillin-resistant gonococci is more than 1%, or unknown, penicillin is not recommended as it is likely to give poor results and may fail to prevent disabling sequelae in some infants. In such a situation, because there is a need for urgent and efficient antibiotic treatment to prevent blindness, a single intramuscular dose of cefotaxime, 100 mg/kg, should be given. This treatment has been successfully used to treat gonococcal conjunctivitis of the newborn, but unfortunately its cost is relatively high. Spectinomycin may be equally efficient, but there is not yet any clinical experience available concerning the use of this drug in the newborn.

Kanamycin has been successfully used to treat gonococcal conjunctivitis in some countries, but its ototoxicity has not yet been sufficiently investigated. A single dose of 25 mg/kg of kanamycin in combination with topical treatment was effective in one study.

If cefotaxime or kanamycin is not available, there may be no alternative to the use of penicillin, but very careful monitoring after treatment is essential. The value of giving higher doses of penicillin in these circumstances has not been studied.

If there is no decrease in the discharge and swelling after 48 hours of systemic treatment, the infant should be referred for further investigation and treatment.

The mother and her partner should receive treatment for gonorrhoea as indicated in Annex 2.

Treatment of presumed chlamydial and other nongonococcal conjunctivitis of the newborn

Infants with onset of infection after 7 days, minimal discharge, and a negative laboratory test for gonococci (if available) should be

5. TREATMENT OF MANIFEST CASES AND EXPOSED INFANTS

treated with topical 1% tetracycline hydrochloride ointment or 0.5% erythromycin ointment 4 times a day for 14 days. For infants with presumed chlamydial conjunctivitis, 50 mg/kg per day of erythromycin syrup should be given by mouth in 4 divided doses for a minimum of 14 days.

Infants exposed to gonorrhoea

Infants known to have been exposed to gonorrhoea at birth should be given full treatment for gonococcal infection, except that topical application of tetracycline hydrochloride ointment can be limited to 4 times a day if there is no conjunctivitis.

6. Health education and training of personnel

Educational needs

Health education may contribute significantly to the prevention of conjunctivitis of the newborn by increasing public awareness of the disease. Such education should involve the whole population, with particular emphasis on future parents. The aims of health education in this context should be (1) to promote awareness and early detection of sexually transmitted diseases; (2) to promote early treatment of sexually transmitted diseases, particularly during pregnancy; and (3) to increase awareness of possible transmission of infection to the newborn, and the consequent risk of blindness.

Cleaning of the eyes of the infant and application of silver nitrate or antibiotic eye ointment immediately after birth should be carefully explained, and the importance of prophylaxis made clear. It is particularly important to influence mothers' attitudes to prophylactic measures if they are to be fully accepted by the local community. Mothers should also be made aware of the need to seek medical care urgently if a child gets red, swollen eyes with discharge, and to comply with the treatment prescribed.

These messages should be understood and actively conveyed by all categories of health personnel, including community health workers and traditional birth attendants. Health education directed against conjunctivitis of the newborn should form part of the overall educational effort and should be conveyed by a wide range of media.

Training needs of health personnel

The implementation of primary health care varies in different countries, and the main training components, given below, should be adapted to the local situation. As a general rule, this training should be practical, directed at the specific tasks to be performed, and should include clear learning objectives. The training should cover:

1. The need for early detection and treatment of sexually transmitted infections in parents, and the risk to newborn

6. HEALTH EDUCATION AND TRAINING OF PERSONNEL

infants. The learning objectives on the prevention and treatment of these conditions will vary according to the background of individual health workers.
2. The application of prophylactic measures in the newborn, i.e., cleaning the eyes and instilling eye drops or applying ointments. It should be explained that a transient chemical conjunctivitis may occur within the first 24 hours after application of silver nitrate.
3. Treatment of manifest cases with combined systemic and topical antibiotics. If systemic antibiotics cannot be administered immediately, primary health care personnel must initiate topical treatment at once and refer the patient for systemic treatment.
4. The need to refer manifest cases of conjunctivitis of the newborn from the community to a referral centre that can provide adequate treatment. It may be necessary to send cases that fail to respond to initial systemic antibiotics direct to a higher level of referral.

Training of personnel in the management of conjunctivitis of the newborn should form part of established basic training schemes for all categories of staff. Refresher courses should be arranged as appropriate to local needs, particularly in view of possible changes in methods of prophylaxis and treatment. Adequate supervision and support from a structured referral system are essential for the management of the disease at the primary health care level. Supervision should include monitoring of the application of preventive measures by birth attendants, and evaluation of treatment and referral of individual cases. Preventive and therapeutic schemes should be improved and modified as appropriate.

Control of conjunctivitis of the newborn can be achieved through a primary health care approach. While all categories of health personnel at the primary level need to be involved in the prevention and management of the disorder, the traditional birth attendants and community health workers have a particularly important role.

7. Logistics of supply of drugs

The following drugs are necessary for the management of conjunctivitis of the newborn: silver nitrate (1%) eye drops, tetracycline hydrochloride (1%) eye ointment, and systemic antibiotics.

Silver nitrate should always be available at the primary health care level, but the solution must be renewed regularly. To avoid evaporation and decomposition during storage, it should be kept in small bottles (2.5 ml) with well-fitting caps; the bottles should be made of dark-coloured glass that is alkali-free or coated with paraffin. Ideally, single-dose preparations of silver nitrate solution should be used, but these are more expensive and are still not widely available.

Silver nitrate can be prepared and distributed at the provincial or district level, provided that satisfactory quality control can be maintained.[1]

Tetracycline hydrochloride (1%) eye ointment is widely available in most countries at a low cost. The preparation is stable, but attention should be paid to its shelf-life.

Antibiotics for the systemic treatment of conjunctivitis of the newborn must be available. In areas with penicillin-resistant strains of *N. gonorrhoeae*, kanamycin or a cephalosporin should be made available. Erythromycin syrup for cases of nongonococcal conjunctivitis should be available at referral level. Antibiotics for the treatment of parents with gonococcal or chlamydial infections must be available, in accordance with national recommendations.

---

[1] *Specifications for the quality control of pharmaceutical preparations: second edition of the International Pharmacopoeia.* Geneva, World Health Organization, 1967, p. 41.

8. Surveillance techniques and reporting

Because of the direct relation between the frequency of maternal gonococcal and chlamydial infections and the incidence of neonatal conjunctivitis, monitoring of pregnant women for sexually transmitted diseases provides an important indicator of the risk of conjunctivitis occurring in the newborn.

National reporting of sexually transmitted diseases varies considerably from country to country; rarely does it go beyond reporting the incidence of syphilis and gonorrhoea, and usually the figures reflect only a fraction of the true occurrence. However, any trends detected are often valid and, as indicators of the risk of conjunctivitis of the newborn, the overall patterns of reported sexually transmitted diseases are pertinent. Reports of cases of conjunctivitis of the newborn from hospitals and clinics, when available, are another important source of information. Hospitals and clinics should be encouraged to separate reports of neonatal conjunctivitis (onset within 28 days of birth or less) from those of all other cases of conjunctivitis.

If available, the results of surveys for sexually transmitted diseases, particularly gonorrhoea, should be examined.

It is important for the pattern of antimicrobial susceptibility of a representative sample of recently isolated gonococcal strains to be examined periodically to detect significant changes in resistance. These patterns may indicate a need for change in the therapeutic regimens recommended for gonococcal infections of adults and of the newborn. At a minimum, the prevalence of penicillinase-producing strains of *N. gonorrhoeae* should be determined.

The outcome of control practices for conjunctivitis of the newborn should be studied whenever possible. In part, this can be achieved by analysing the number of infants that present at district hospitals because initial treatment has failed or the condition has recurred, and the number with severe corneal damage and/or blindness—these represent the failure of the control strategy. The occurrence of neonatal conjunctivitis in different population groups should be continuously monitored to assess the efficacy of prophylactic strategies and the magnitude of the problem. Where facilities are available, sample surveys should be carried out, and repeated at intervals, to assess the incidence of conjunctivitis of the newborn and changes in the relative frequency of the different causes.

Sample surveys of pregnant women should be conducted to establish the prevalence of gonococcal infection and, when possible, the relative frequency of antibiotic-resistant strains. Sampling should take into account significant factors such as social class, ethnic group, rural or urban origin, etc. In most instances, such surveys will have to be restricted to studies of gonococcal prevalence alone, but when laboratory facilities are available the prevalence of *C. trachomatis* should also be evaluated.

Acknowledgements

The colour photographs were kindly supplied by Dr A. Meheus, University of Antwerp, Wilrijk, Belgium; Dr P. Rapoza, The Wilmer Institute, The Johns Hopkins School of Hygiene and Public Health, Baltimore, MD, USA; Dr M. Valenton, Philippine Eye Research Institute, Manila, Philippines; and Dr F. Yvert, Centre international de Recherches médicales, Franceville, Gabon.

Summary

The worldwide increase in the incidence of gonorrhoea has resulted in a corresponding increase in gonococcal conjunctivitis of the newborn. The situation has been made worse by the premature abandonment of prophylactic measures in some countries. Gonococcal conjunctivitis of the newborn is a serious blinding condition that can easily be prevented; ocular prophylaxis of the newborn is therefore an essential part of primary health care.

Gonococcal conjunctivitis of the newborn can be prevented by identifying and treating pregnant women with gonorrhoea and their sexual partners, and by applying prophylactic medication to the eyes of infants immediately after birth. Because routine detection of gonorrhoea during pregnancy is rarely possible, prophylactic treatment of newborn infants is the main means of prevention. Prophylaxis in the newborn consists of cleaning the eyelids and applying either 1 % silver nitrate drops or 1 % tetracycline hydrochloride ointment to the eyes as soon as possible after delivery. It is particularly important to carry out prophylaxis wherever there is a high prevalence of gonococcal infection in adults.

With the increasing prevalence of penicillin-resistant strains of *Neisseria gonorrhoeae*, penicillin is no longer the only antibiotic recommended for the treatment of gonococcal conjunctivitis of the newborn. Where the prevalence of penicillin-resistant strains is known to be above 1 %, alternative antimicrobial agents should be used; several suitable antibiotics are available, and treatment schedules are recommended. Treatment with systemic and topical antimicrobial agents must be started as early as possible to preserve sight. The management of neonatal conjunctivitis caused by *Chlamydia trachomatis* is also discussed.

Prevention and management of gonococcal conjunctivitis of the newborn should ideally be the responsibility of primary health care workers, but it is important that all personnel involved in the delivery and care of infants should be able to apply ocular prophylaxis, recognize gonococcal conjunctivitis, and initiate appropriate treatment.

Annex 1

Laboratory methods used for identifying causes of conjunctivitis of the newborn

This annex explains how to obtain specimens from the eye and gives details of the laboratory techniques used to identify conjunctivitis of the newborn caused by *Neisseria gonorrhoeae*, *Chlamydia trachomatis*, and other bacteria.

Microscopic examination of stained slides

Specimen collection

Exudate smears. Microscopic examination of stained smears of discharge from the eye is a sensitive and specific method of diagnosing gonococcal conjunctivitis of the newborn. Material from the eye is obtained by pulling down the lower lid and gently rubbing a dry cotton swab or spatula over the surface of the exposed conjunctiva. This exudate should then be spread in a thin layer on a clean glass slide and air-dried. Ideally the specimen should be fixed immediately, but if this is not possible fixation should not be delayed for more than a few hours.

Conjunctival scrapings. Conjunctivitis of the newborn caused by *C. trachomatis* can be diagnosed by microscopic examination of intact epithelial cells. Whole cells are obtained by using a spatula with a fine (but not sharp) edge to scrape the exposed surface of the conjunctiva, using firm even strokes; the spatula should be held perpendicular to the surface of the conjunctiva. Standard Lindner or Kimura spatulas are suitable for this purpose, but if these are not available a similar spatula can be made by flattening one end of a thin aluminium rod until the tip is about 3 mm wide.

The material scraped from the conjunctiva should be spread thinly

ANNEX 1

on to a clean glass slide and then air-dried and fixed as soon as possible. Once fixed, slides may be stored for several days before being stained. Slides for immunofluorescent staining should be stored at −20°C.

Staining[1]

Smears of exudate should be stained with Gram stain or methylene blue, and examined under a microscope. Smears are positive for *N. gonorrhoeae* if typical Gram-negative diplococci are found within polymorphonuclear leukocytes; equivocal or inconclusive if extracellular Gram-negative diplococci are present; and negative if diplococci are not found. Infants with an equivocal or inconclusive smear test should nevertheless be treated for gonococcal conjunctivitis.

To identify intracytoplasmic inclusions of *C. trachomatis* in smears of conjunctival scrapings, Giemsa stain should be used. Alternative stains that give reasonable results are Wright stain and Dif-Kwik. Other stains, such as Papanicolaou, are unsatisfactory.

A stock solution of Giemsa stain can be prepared by dissolving 0.5 g of powdered stain in 33 ml of glycerol at 55–60°C for 1½–2 hours; 33 ml of acetone-free, absolute methanol should then be added and the mixture stirred thoroughly. The solution should be left for a few hours for the sediment to settle, and then filtered.

An alternative method of preparing a stock solution is to mix 0.75 g of powdered Giemsa stain with 35 ml of glycerol and 65 ml of absolute methanol in a bottle containing glass beads. The bottle should be shaken 3 times a day for 4 days. The solution should then be filtered into a clean bottle. The stock solution of Giemsa stain must be stored in the dark.

Fresh Giemsa stain should be prepared daily by adding 1 part of the stock solution to 40 or 50 parts of neutral distilled water. The solution should be filtered before use. The fresh stain should only be used for one day.

It is essential that the distilled water used for diluting the stock solution of stain has a pH between 6.8 and 7.2; this is achieved by adding standard phosphate buffer. Standard phosphate buffer consists of: (*a*) a 0.067 mol/litre solution of disodium hydrogen phosphate, prepared by dissolving 9.5 g of Na_2HPO_4 in a small amount of distilled water and then making the volume up to 1 litre by adding more distilled water; and (*b*) a 0.067 mol/litre solution of sodium dihydrogen phosphate, prepared by dissolving 9.2 g of NaH_2PO_4 in

---

[1] Details on the preparation of stains and other reagents are given in the *Manual of basic techniques for a health laboratory*. Geneva, World Health Organization, 1980, pp. 465–477.

distilled water using the same method as for solution (a).

Buffered water, pH 7.2, is obtained by mixing 72 ml of solution (a) with 28 ml of solution (b) and adding 900 ml of distilled water. This solution should be filtered before use.

Before Giemsa staining, smears should be fixed for 5 minutes in absolute methanol and then air-dried. To stain the smears, the slides are immersed or covered with Giemsa stain for 1 hour, and then rinsed rapidly with 95% ethanol to remove excess stain. After air-drying, the preparations are permanent and can be examined with a light microscope.

The appearance of chlamydial inclusions in conjunctival epithelial cells is described in several publications.[1,2,3]

Presumptive identification of bacteria can also be made in Giemsa-stained conjunctival smears.

The use of immunofluorescent stains, fluorescein conjugated immune serum or monoclonal antibody, or the iodine stain to detect chlamydial inclusions in conjunctival smears of the newborn appears to have little advantage over conventional Giemsa stain.

The sensitivity of the Giemsa stain for detecting chlamydial conjunctivitis of the newborn is equal to that of cell culture or immunofluorescent staining. This is not true for conjunctivitis in older children and adults, or for chlamydial genital infection, where culture and immunofluorescent methods are considerably more sensitive. Microscopic examination of Giemsa-stained conjunctival smears is the best method of diagnosing chlamydial conjunctivitis of the newborn because of its simplicity, excellent sensitivity and specificity, and widespread availability.

Culture of *N. gonorrhoeae*[4]

A variety of media can be used to culture *N. gonorrhoeae* including modified Thayer-Martin medium, New York City medium, enriched chocolate agar (e.g., Isovitalex[5]), or sheep's blood agar (human blood agar is not suitable).

To obtain a sample from the eye for culture, the conjunctival

---

[1] *Guide to the laboratory diagnosis of trachoma.* Geneva, World Health Organization, 1975.

[2] Schachter, J. & Dawson, C. R. *Human chlamydial infections.* Littleton, Publishing Sciences Group, 1978.

[3] Yoneda, C., et al. Cytology as a guide to the presence of chlamydial inclusions in Giemsa-stained conjunctival smears in severe trachoma. *British journal of ophthalmology,* **59**: 116–124 (1975).

[4] WHO Technical Report Series, No. 616, 1978 (Neisseria gonorrhoeae and gonococcal infections: report of a WHO Scientific Group).

[5] Produced by Baltimore Biological Laboratories, Cockeysville, MD, USA.

surface should be rubbed directly with a cotton swab moistened with sterile water, sterile saline, or sterile broth. Ideally the culture medium (which should be at room temperature) should be streaked immediately with the swab; if this is not possible the sample should be transferred to a solid transport medium such as Transgrow[1] or, alternatively, the entire swab can be stored in a semi-solid transport medium such as Stuart medium. The use of dry swabs or the storage or transport of swabs in a dry sterile tube will result in lower rates of recovery from infected eyes.

Once inoculated, plates should be incubated as soon as possible in a candle jar, a plastic bag containing carbon dioxide generating tablets, or a carbon dioxide incubator (5–10% CO_2, 50–70% relative humidity). The best temperature for incubating *N. gonorrhoeae* is 35–36°C.

The media should be examined 24 and 48 hours after inoculation for colonies. On primary isolation on Thayer-Martin plates, gonococcal colonies are moderately convex, greyish-white, glistening, and finely granular; suspect colonies can be identified by smear and the oxidase test. Oxidase-positive isolates from the eye that grow on a selective medium do not need to be confirmed as *N. gonorrhoeae*. Eventual confirmation of isolates can be done by sugar degradation tests.[2]

---

[1] See footnote 1 on page 11.
[2] See footnote 4 on page 26.

Annex 2
Therapeutic recommendations for treatment of gonococcal infections in adults[1]

Uncomplicated urogenital infection

Group A

The following regimens remain useful in areas in which gonococci are known to have maintained chromosomal sensitivity to antimicrobial agents and penicillinase-producing strains of gonococci comprise less than 1 % of isolates:

- amoxicillin, 3.0 g, with 1.0 g of probenecid by mouth, or
- ampicillin, 3.5 g, with 1.0 g of probenecid by mouth, or
- procaine benzylpenicillin, 4.8 g (4.8 million units) by intramuscular injection, with 1.0 g of probenecid by mouth, or
- benzylpenicillin, 3.0 g (5 million units) by intramuscular injection, with 1.0 g of probenecid by mouth, or
- tetracycline hydrochloride, 500 mg by mouth, 4 times a day for 7 days, or
- doxycycline hydrochloride, 100 mg by mouth, twice daily for 7 days.

Group B

In areas where the chromosomal resistance of gonococci has reduced the efficacy of antimicrobial agents such as benzylpenicillin,

---

[1] From the report of the WHO Expert Committee on Venereal Diseases and Treponematoses, 1–7 November 1983 (WHO Technical Report Series, in press). These recommendations are subject to periodical amendments.

tetracycline, and sulfamethoxazole + trimethoprim to below 95%, and in areas where penicillinase-producing gonococci are prevalent, the following single-session regimens remain effective in at least 95% of cases:

spectinomycin, 2.0 g by intramuscular injection, or

cefotaxime, 1.0 g by intramuscular injection, or

cefoxitin, 2.0 g by intramuscular injection, with 1.0 g of probenecid by mouth, or

ceftriaxone, 250 mg by intramuscular injection.

Group C

The following regimens that are effective against penicillinase-producing gonococci show considerable geographic variation in their efficacy, sometimes curing less than 95% of infections:

kanamycin, 2.0 g by intramuscular injection, or
thiamphenicol, 2.5 g by mouth, or

sulfamethoxazole (400 mg) + trimethoprim (80 mg), 10 tablets by mouth daily for 3 days.

Annex 3
List of participants

Dr C. R. Dawson, Francis I. Proctor Foundation for Research in Ophthalmology, University of California, San Francisco, CA, USA (*Rapporteur*)
Dr P. Mansuwan, Director, The Children's Hospital, Bangkok, Thailand
Dr A. Meheus, University of Antwerp, Epidemiology and Social Medicine, Universiteitsplein 1, Wilrijk, Belgium (*Chairman*)
Dr J. D. Oriel, Department of Genito-Urinary Medicine, University College Hospital, Gower Street, London, England
Professor C. O. Quarcoopome, WHO Consultant for Prevention of Blindness in Africa, Lilongwe, Malawi
Dr K. V. Trutneva, Director, Helmholtz Research Institute of Ophthalmology, Moscow, USSR
Dr M. Valenton, Philippine Eye Research Institute, Philippine General Hospital Compound, Manila, Philippines

WHO Secretariat
Dr G. Antal, Bacterial and Venereal Infections, WHO, Geneva, Switzerland
Dr G. Causse, Bacterial and Venereal Infections, WHO, Geneva, Switzerland
Dr J. F. Dunne, Pharmaceuticals, WHO, Geneva, Switzerland
Dr D. Flahault, Health Team Development, WHO, Geneva, Switzerland
Dr T. Kereselidze, Bacterial and Venereal Infections, WHO, Geneva, Switzerland
Dr K. Konyama, Programme for the Prevention of Blindness, WHO, Geneva, Switzerland
Ms E. Leedham, Consultant, Maternal and Child Health, WHO, Geneva, Switzerland
Dr R. Pararajasegaram, Regional Adviser for the Prevention of Blindness, WHO Regional Office for South-East Asia, New Delhi, India

ANNEX 3

Dr B. Thylefors, Programme for the Prevention of Blindness, WHO, Geneva, Switzerland

Dr G. Vartanian, Office of Research Promotion and Development, WHO, Geneva, Switzerland

WHO publications may be obtained, direct or through booksellers, from:

ALGERIA: Entreprise...
ARGENTINA: Carlos...
AUSTRALIA: Hunter... Government Publishing Service (Mail order sales),... Government Publishing Service Bookshops at; 70 A... ensland 4000; 347 Swanston Street, MELBOURN... eorge's Terrace, PERTH, WA 6000; Industry Ho... S 7000 — R. Hill & Son Ltd., 608 St. Kilda Road... NSW 2065
AUSTRIA: Gerold...
BAHRAIN: United...
BANGLADESH: Th...
BELGIUM: For book... eriodicals and subscriptions: Office International... lth only: Jean de Lannoy, 202 avenue du Roi, 10...
BHUTAN: see India...
BOTSWANA: Bots...
BRAZIL: Biblioteca... .381, Vila Clementino, 04023 SÃO PAULO, S.P....
BURMA: see India,...
CANADA: Canadian... 8N8. (Tel: (613) 725–3769. Telex: 21-053-384...
CHINA: China Nati...
CYPRUS: "MAM",...
CZECHOSLOVAKIA...
DEMOCRATIC PEO...
DENMARK: Munks... (Tel: + 45 1 12 85 70)
ECUADOR: Libreria...
EGYPT: Osiris Offic...
FIJI: The WHO Pro...
FINLAND: Akateem...
FRANCE: Librairie...
GABON: Librairie U...
GERMAN DEMOCR...
GERMANY FEDERA... 6236 ESCHBORN — W. E. Saarbach GmbH, T... hhandlung Alexander Horn, Friedrichstrasse 39,... PRINTED IN U.S.A.
GHANA: Fides Ente...
GREECE: G.C. Eleftheroudakis S.A., Librairie internationale, rue Nikis 4, ATHENS (T. 126)
HAITI: Max Bouchereau, Librairie "A la Caravelle", Boîte postale III-B, P-PRINCE
HONG KONG: Hong Kong Government Information Services, Beaconsfield House, 6th Floor, Queen's Road, Central, VICTORIA
HUNGARY: Kultura, P.O.B. 149, BUDAPEST 62 — Akadémiai Könyvesbolt, Váci utca 22, BUDAPEST V
ICELAND: Snaebjørn Jonsson & Co., P.O. Box 1131, Hafnarstraeti 9, REYKJAVIK
INDIA: WHO Regional Office for South-East Asia, World Health House, Indraprastha Estate, Mahatma Gandhi Road, NEW DELHI 110002
INDONESIA: P.T. Kalman Media Pusaka, Pusat Perdagangan Senen, Block I, 4th Floor, P.O. Box 3433/Jkt, JAKARTA
IRAN (ISLAMIC REPUBLIC OF): Iran University Press, 85 Park Avenue, P.O. Box 54/551, TEHERAN
IRAQ: Ministry of Information, National House for Publishing, Distributing and Advertising, BAGHDAD
IRELAND: TDC Publishers, 12 North Frederick Street, DUBLIN 1 (Tel: 744835–749677)
ISRAEL: Heiliger & Co., 3 Nathan Strauss Street, JERUSALEM 94227
ITALY: Edizioni Minerva Medica, Corso Bramante 83–85, 10126 TURIN; Via Lamarmora 3, 20100 MILAN
JAPAN: Maruzen Co. Ltd., P.O. Box 5050, TOKYO International, 100–31
JORDAN: Jordan Book Centre Co. Ltd., University Street, P.O. Box 301 (Al-Jubeiha), AMMAN
KUWAIT: The Kuwait Bookshops Co. Ltd., Thunayan Al-Ghanem Bldg, P.O. Box 2942, KUWAIT
LAOS PEOPLE'S DEMOCRATIC REPUBLIC: The WHO Programme Coordinator, P.O. Box 343, VIENTIANE
LEBANON: The Levant Distributors Co. S.A.R.L., Box 1181, Makdassi Street, Hanna Bldg, BEIRUT
LUXEMBOURG: Librairie du Centre, 49 bd Royal, LUXEMBOURG
MALAWI: Malawi Book Service, P.O. Box 30044, Chichiti, BLANTYRE 3

A/I/85